I0697484

SURVIVING URINARY INCONTINENCE

Beginners Comprehensive Approach To Combating & Managing Urinary Incontinence Outbreak Effectively

Nuel Nenji

Copyright © 2023 By Nuel Nenji

All Rights Reserved

Table of Contents

Introductory

When a person is unable to control their bladder, they may experience involuntary urination, sometimes known as "leaking." This medical condition is known as urinary incontinence. Mild cases include those where urination occurs only seldom, such as while coughing or sneezing, whereas severe cases involve a total loss of bladder control.

Symptoms of urinary incontinence range from:

• Coughing, sneezing, laughing, or vigorous exercise can all cause a form of incontinence known as stress incontinence. Weak pelvic floor muscles have been associated to this condition.

• Overactive bladder, or urge incontinence, is characterized by an abrupt and strong need to urinate followed by the involuntary loss of urine. One possible cause is a detrusor muscle in the bladder that is overly active.

• When the bladder is unable to empty completely, a condition known as overflow incontinence sets in. This is characterized by the involuntary passage of small volumes of pee. Causes include urinary tract blockage, nerve injury, and some pharmaceuticals.

• Physical or mental impairments can make it difficult to get to the bathroom in time, leading to functional incontinence that is unrelated to bladder or urinary system dysfunction.

• Some people, called those with "mixed incontinence," struggle with both stress and urge incontinence at the same time.

Although urinary incontinence can occur at any age, it most frequently affects the elderly, particularly women who have given birth or gone through menopause. Treatment methods range from behavioral modification and pelvic floor exercises (Kegel exercises) to pharmaceuticals, medical technologies, and even surgical intervention. Treatment for incontinence should be determined in collaboration with a medical professional and is condition-specific.

CHAPTER ONE
Structure And Function Of The Male And Female Urinary Systems

The urinary system, also called the renal system, is responsible for producing and excreting urine, which the body uses to flush out waste products and excess substances from the circulatory system.

A network of organs and tissues, it coordinates the body's efforts to regulate fluid and electrolyte levels. The urinary system's anatomy and physiology are summarized below.

1. Kidneys:

• The kidneys, which are about the size of a bean, sit on either side of the spine, below the rib cage.

• Urine is produced when waste items, extra ions (such potassium and sodium), and water are filtered out of the blood.

• To create urine, the kidneys use specialized cells called nephrons to filter and digest blood.

2. Ureters:

• The kidneys are linked to the bladder via two tubes called ureters, one from each kidney.

• They use peristaltic contractions to move urine from the kidneys to the bladder.

3. Bladder, Urinary:

• Urine is held in the urinary bladder, a muscular sac, until it can be released from the body.

• It may extend to store a wide range of urine volumes and is situated in the pelvis.

4. Urethra:

• The urethra connects the urinary bladder to the outside world.

• During ejaculation, a man's semen travels through the urethra.

The Body's Mechanics:

The urinary system is responsible for a number of important physiological processes, including:

• The kidneys are responsible for filtering the blood and excreting any unwanted substances, including waste products (such urea and creatinine), excess ions, and water, in the form of urine. This process aids in homeostasis by controlling the levels of numerous chemicals in the blood.

• The kidneys help control blood pressure by modifying plasma volume and by secreting the enzyme renin.

• The urinary system plays an important role in maintaining the body's electrolyte balance by flushing out excess sodium, potassium, calcium, and phosphate.

• The acid-base balance of the body is maintained by the kidneys, which excrete hydrogen ions and reabsorb bicarbonate ions, respectively.

• In reaction to low oxygen levels in the blood, the kidneys manufacture and secrete the hormone erythropoietin, which stimulates the creation of red blood cells.

• The elimination of toxins, medications, and foreign substances through the urinary system is an important part of the detoxification process.

• The kidneys aid in maintaining a healthy water balance by regulating how much water is reabsorbed into the bloodstream and how much is expelled in urine.

The urinary system plays a crucial role in the body's maintenance of homeostasis, as it is responsible for the efficient removal of waste products and the regulation of many vital bodily functions.

Reasons And Potential Threats

Causes and risk factors for urinary incontinence might vary from one kind of the condition to another. The following are some of the most common causes and risk factors of urine incontinence:

1. Incontinence due to Stress:

• The pelvic floor muscles are stretched and weakened during pregnancy and vaginal deliveries, which can lead to stress incontinence.

• Stress incontinence is more common in older adults because the muscles and tissues that support the bladder may deteriorate.

• Obesity is a risk factor for stress incontinence because it increases strain on the pelvic floor and bladder.

• Intense strain on the pelvic floor muscles, such as those caused by smoking or respiratory issues, can result in stress incontinence.

• The risk of developing stress incontinence is increased by actions like heavy lifting and straining that are performed on a regular basis.

2. The Need to Go Potty:

• Overactive Bladder (OAB): People with this disorder have sudden and strong needs to urinate. However, nerve issues, bladder irritation, and other medical diseases can all contribute to OAB, making it difficult to pinpoint a single, definitive reason.

• Neurological disorders can cause urge incontinence by interfering with the normal functioning of the nerves that control the bladder. These disorders include multiple sclerosis, stroke, and spinal cord damage.

Infections, bladder stones, and some medications can all irritate the bladder and lead to the need to urinate frequently and urgently.

3. Incontinence of Excess Fluids:

• An enlarged prostate in men is just one condition that can obstruct the urethra and cause overflow incontinence in women.

• Diabetes, spinal cord injuries, and other neurological illnesses can all cause nerve damage, which can in turn impair the bladder's capacity to contract and empty properly.

4. Irregular Bladder Function:

• Physical restrictions, such as arthritis, severe joint pain, or cognitive difficulties, might make it difficult to get to the bathroom in time, which can lead to functional incontinence.

5. Uneven Bladder Leakage:

• It can be more difficult to identify the root cause of mixed incontinence because it typically involves more than one of the aforementioned categories of incontinence.

CHAPTER TWO
Predisposing Factors For Incontinence Of Urination

The aging process and the resulting weakening of the pelvic floor muscles greatly enhance the likelihood of urine incontinence in older adults.

• Gender: Pregnancy, childbirth, and menopause put women at a higher risk for urine incontinence than males do.

• Obesity: Being overweight plays a role in both stress and urge incontinence.

• Stress incontinence may develop as a result of the constant coughing that is a side effect of smoking.

• Some people may have a higher risk of developing urine incontinence due to a family history of the condition.

• Urinary incontinence is more likely to occur in people with certain medical conditions, such as diabetes, persistent constipation, and chronic respiratory disorders.

It's crucial to remember that each person's experience with urine incontinence will be unique, and that some may have a combination of risk factors. Urinary incontinence can be embarrassing and uncomfortable, so it's best to get it checked out by a doctor if you or someone you know is having problems with it.

Symptoms

Depending on the cause, a person may experience a wide range of different urine incontinence symptoms. The most prevalent forms of urine incontinence are characterized by the following symptoms:

1. Incontinence due to Stress:

• Stress incontinence sufferers may have accidents when they do things that exert stress on their bladder, like lifting heavy objects, exercising, laughing, or sneezing.

• Stress incontinence is characterized by the rapid and involuntary loss of control over the release of a small amount of pee.

• Stress incontinence sufferers, in contrast to those who suffer from urge incontinence, do not typically feel an urgent need to urinate just before any leakage occurs.

2. The Need to Go Potty:

• People who suffer from urge incontinence frequently struggle to control sudden, intense desires to urinate.

• There may be a frequent need to urinate even if the bladder is not full.

• When the need to urinate is too great to ignore or when there isn't enough time to get to the bathroom, urine leakage can occur.

• Most people with urge incontinence have very little or no notice before they start to leak.

3. Incontinence of Excess Fluids:

• Frequent dribbling: People with overflow incontinence may leak little amounts of pee repeatedly throughout the day and night.

• They may have trouble urinating all the way to the toilet because they have trouble emptying their bladder.

• Weak or Intermittent Urine Flow: The flow of urine may be weak or sporadic.

4. Irregular Bladder Function:

Functional incontinence is distinguished from other forms of incontinence by the following symptoms.

• Delayed Toilet Use: People with functional incontinence may have difficulties reaching the toilet in time due to physical or cognitive limitations, but they may not suffer from bladder or sphincter disorders.

They may recognize the need to urinate yet be unable to reach the restroom without assistance.

5. Uneven Bladder Leakage:

Mixed incontinence occurs when symptoms of both stress incontinence and urge incontinence coexist. Symptoms of stress and urge incontinence, for instance, may coexist in the same individual.

Urinary incontinence is very frequent, and the intensity of its symptoms varies greatly from person to person. Some people may only have mild, infrequent leakage, while others may have severe, chronic symptoms that severely limit their daily activities.

Urinary incontinence is a medical condition that should be evaluated and treated if symptoms are present. Depending on the kind and severity of incontinence, a healthcare practitioner can diagnose the underlying reason and propose a course of treatment, which may involve dietary and behavioral modifications, physical therapy, medication, or even surgery.

CHAPTER THREE
Testing For Incontinence Of Urination

Urinary incontinence is usually diagnosed after a comprehensive medical evaluation by a doctor. These possible steps are included in the process:

1.The first step in treating incontinence is for the doctor to get a thorough understanding of the patient's medical history, asking questions about the patient's urine symptoms, the frequency and intensity of incontinence episodes, any triggering factors (such as coughing or sneezing), and the impact incontinence has on the patient's daily life. They will also ask about past medical history, current treatment, and lifestyle choices.

2. In order to determine if there are any underlying physical causes for incontinence, a thorough physical examination should be performed. The doctor may check for signs of infection or neurological disorders, as well as evaluate the patient's pelvic floor muscles' strength.

3. Keeping a bladder diary can be helpful in understanding one's urination patterns. Patients may be required to keep diaries for many days to track things like fluid intake, urination frequency, and urinary leakage.

4. An analysis of a urine sample for the presence of infection, blood, or other abnormalities that could be causing urinary symptoms is called a urinalysis.

5. Measuring the volume of pee still present in the bladder after urination is one way to evaluate bladder emptying when it is indicated. Ultrasound or catheterization can be used for this purpose.

6. Urodynamic Testing: These tests are more in-depth evaluations of bladder and urine function than regular exams. These examinations may consist of:

• Cystometry is a test that measures the bladder's capacity and pressure as it fills with fluid.

• Uroflowmetry is a technique used to gauge the speed with which a person urinates.

• Voiding-specific pressure and flow studies assess bladder and urethral function.

7. Imaging techniques, such as ultrasonography, cystoscopy, or magnetic resonance imaging, may be

performed to assess urinary tract structure and function.

8. A neurological evaluation of nerve function may be undertaken if it is considered that neurological disorders are the root cause of urine incontinence.

9. Additional specialist testing may be required to determine the incontinence subtype and etiology, depending on the patient's clinical presentation.

10.Patients may be asked to fill out questionnaires or other assessment instruments to gauge the extent to which incontinence affects their daily lives.

After gathering all the necessary data, a doctor can diagnose incontinence based on the specific kind (stress, urge, mixed) and the etiology (pregnancy, neurological illness, etc.). The patient's unique needs can then be assessed, and a treatment plan developed accordingly.

Communicating clearly and honestly with your doctor about your symptoms and medical history is essential for getting a proper diagnosis and designing a suitable treatment plan.

Seeking medical help is crucial if you're dealing with urine incontinence so you can improve your quality of life, since many cases may be successfully controlled or treated.

Choices In Medical Care

Urinary incontinence can be treated in a number of ways, but the specifics of those methods are condition- and cause-specific. Conservative and non-invasive techniques are one option, while more invasive therapies are another. Urinary incontinence typically responds to the following treatments:

1. Interventions in Lifestyle and Behavior:

• Kegel exercises, which target the pelvic floor muscles, can assist those with stress incontinence and even some cases of mixed incontinence regain control of their bladders.

• Bladder training is a method used to treat urge incontinence that entails urinating at regular intervals and gradually increasing the time between bathroom trips.

• Urinary symptoms can be alleviated by changing fluid intake and decreasing caffeine and alcohol use, especially in the evening.

• Avoiding bladder-irritating foods and drinks (such spicy foods and fizzy drinks) may help with dietary changes.

• If you're overweight, losing weight can help by putting less strain on your bladder and pelvic floor.

• To reduce the risk of stress incontinence, it is recommended that smokers quit.

2. Medications:

• Urge incontinence is typically treated with anticholinergic or antispasmodic drugs, which help relax the hyperactive bladder muscles and lessen the need to urinate frequently or frequently.

• Postmenopausal women may be offered estrogen therapy to help increase tissue tone and alleviate symptoms of stress incontinence.

3. Surgical Instruments:

• Pessaries are vaginally inserted devices used to treat stress incontinence and pelvic organ prolapse by providing bladder support and reducing the risk of urine leakage.

• Urethral Inserts: These are tiny devices that are put into the urethra before engaging in activities that may cause incontinence.

4. Stimulating the Nerves:

• Implanting a device that provides electrical impulses to the sacral nerves (which regulate bladder function) is known as sacral nerve stimulation (InterStim). It's useful for managing overactive bladder and urge incontinence.

5. Treatment Via Injections:

Overactive bladder muscles can be temporarily relaxed and urge incontinence symptoms reduced by injecting Botulinum toxin (Botox) into the bladder wall.

6. Surgery:

• Stress incontinence can be treated using sling procedures, which involve surgically inserting a sling or mesh to support the urethra or bladder neck.

• Stress incontinence is a typical reason for bladder neck suspension, a treatment that stabilizes the urethra and bladder neck.

• The artificial urinary sphincter is a device used to treat severe cases of stress incontinence by opening and closing the urethra through surgical implantation and manual control.

• Stress incontinence is commonly treated by colposuspension, a surgical procedure that suspends the urethra and bladder.

7. Medical Interventions:

• To treat stress incontinence and enhance urethral closure, bulking agents can be injected into the tissues surrounding the urethra.

The incontinence type, its intensity, the patient's general health, and the patient's preferences all play a role in determining the best course of treatment.

The best course of treatment should be determined after discussion with a medical professional. Urinary incontinence is often treated with a multifaceted strategy that may involve behavioral modification, pelvic floor exercises, and medication.

CHAPTER FOUR
Care For Incontinence Of Urination

There is no single cure for urine incontinence, but a mix of treatments can help alleviate symptoms and restore independence. The incontinence's intensity and cause will determine the best method of treatment. Some overarching methods for dealing with urine incontinence are as follows:

1. Interventions in Lifestyle and Behavior:

• Kegel exercises, which target the pelvic floor muscles, can assist those with stress incontinence and even some cases of mixed incontinence regain control of their bladders. The pelvic floor muscles are worked by contracting and then relaxing. It's important to get them right, so checking in with a doctor or physical therapist might help.

• Bladder training is a method for improving the amount of time you can go without needing to urinate. Extend the time you wait to urinate by 10–15 minutes to start, then go from there.

• Controlling fluid and food intake can help people urinate less frequently, especially at night. Caffeine, alcohol, and spicy foods can all irritate the bladder and should be avoided.

• If you are overweight, lowering weight may help alleviate symptoms by reducing the strain on your bladder and pelvic floor muscles.

• Smoking contributes to chronic coughing, which can exacerbate other symptoms. Stress incontinence may improve if you give up smoking.

2. Medications:

• The urgency and frequency of urine can be reduced by using anticholinergic or antispasmodic medication, which is commonly prescribed for people with urge incontinence.

• Postmenopausal women may be offered estrogen therapy to help increase tissue tone and alleviate symptoms of stress incontinence.

3. Products for Incontinence:

• To prevent discomfort and preserve your privacy, use absorbent materials such as adult diapers, pads, or liners.

4. Pilates for the Pelvic Floor:

• A pelvic floor physical therapist can help you strengthen and better coordinate your pelvic floor muscles with targeted exercises and techniques.

5. Interventions in Behavior:

• Create a routine for when you urinate to teach your bladder to empty at certain times.

• The bladder can be emptied more thoroughly if you "double void" by urinating, waiting a few minutes, and then urinating again.

6. Inserts for the Urethra and Pessaries:

• Symptoms can be alleviated and bladder support improved with the help of a pessary (a device put into the vagina) or urethral implant for some women.

7. Stimulating the Nerves:

• Surgical implantation of a device that transmits electrical impulses to the sacral nerves (InterStim) to improve bladder control. It's useful for managing overactive bladder and urge incontinence.

8. Injectable Botox:

• Overactive bladder muscles can be relaxed and urge incontinence symptoms mitigated using Botulinum toxin (Botox) injections into the bladder wall.

9. Surgery Choices:

• Sling installation, bladder neck suspension, artificial urinary sphincter implantation, and colposuspension are some of the surgical techniques that may be considered, depending on the kind and severity of incontinence.

10. Interventions to Help:

• If you're struggling to deal with incontinence, joining a support group or seeing a counselor can help.

You and your doctor should collaborate together to create a treatment strategy that is just right for you. The various methods of treating urine incontinence may be combined in many patients. With proper care, incontinence can have much less of an effect on your daily life, greatly enhancing your quality of life.

Preventative Medicine And The Future

The prognosis for urine incontinence and the likelihood that it can be prevented depends on a number of factors, such as the nature and origins of the condition. While some risk factors for urinary incontinence, such age and genetics, may be out of your control, there are things you can do to lower your risk and enhance your bladder health.

1. Abdominal Strengthening:

• Strengthening the muscles that support the bladder and regulate urine flow can be accomplished by performing pelvic floor muscle exercises (Kegel exercises) on a regular basis. Stress incontinence is one type of incontinence that may be alleviated with these exercises.

2. Keeping a Healthy BMI

• Reduce stress on your bladder and pelvic floor muscles by getting to and staying at a healthy weight. If you are overweight, losing weight can help you avoid or manage incontinence.

3. Consume Plenty of Water and a Well-Rounded Diet:

• Hydrate regularly during the day, but watch your fluid intake in the hours before bed to cut down on bathroom trips.

• Constipation, which can worsen urinary incontinence, can be avoided by eating a diet high in fiber.

4. Keep Your Bladder Stress-Free:

• Caffeine, alcohol, spicy meals, and citrus fruits may all aggravate bladder irritation and should be avoided or consumed in moderation.

5. Quitting Smoking:

• If you want to avoid stress incontinence and a chronic cough, you should stop smoking.

6. Control Long-Term Illness:

• In order to prevent nerve damage and other issues that might lead to incontinence, people with chronic diseases like diabetes should keep their blood sugar levels under tight control.

7. Maintaining Proper Bathroom Hygiene:

• Don't be in a hurry to use the restroom; instead, take the time to urinate thoroughly.

• Don't put stress on your pelvic floor muscles by squeezing when you have to go to the bathroom.

8. Keeping Busy:

• Consistent exercise is recommended for incontinence prevention and general health maintenance.

9. Stop smoking and get medical help if you have a persistent cough from another cause; this will help reduce the strain on your pelvic floor muscles.

10. The risk of pelvic floor injury can be reduced by using specific delivery procedures, which you and your healthcare practitioner can discuss if you are planning a pregnancy.

The prognosis for people who suffer from urine incontinence is bright. In many cases, treatment or management can significantly reduce symptoms and enhance quality of life.

The diagnosis and treatment of urine incontinence have both benefited greatly from recent medical advances.

Urinary incontinence is a medical emergency that has to be treated as soon as possible. Preventing the problem from getting worse and giving you more options to meet your individual requirements is the goal of early intervention.

Many people will be able to experience better bladder health and less symptoms of incontinence in the future if they receive the appropriate care and make the necessary changes to their lifestyle.

Conclusion

Uncontrollable urination is a frequent medical disorder known as urinary incontinence. A proper diagnosis and therapy can help many people regain bladder control and alleviate their symptoms, greatly improving their quality of life.

For successful care, it is essential to identify the specific kind and underlying reasons of urine incontinence. Depending on the severity of the condition, medical professionals may recommend medication, medical devices, or even surgery in addition to lifestyle and behavioral therapies including pelvic floor exercises and dietary adjustments.

You can lessen your chances of developing incontinence by taking precautions, like living a healthy lifestyle, using your bladder properly, and getting treatment for any underlying chronic problems that could be causing your symptoms.

Improvements in treatment and research have led to an optimistic outlook for people living with urine incontinence. Many people can benefit from improved bladder health and an increased quality of life with the help of professional supervision and proactive management of the problem.

Seek professional help and learn about your treatment options if you or someone you know has urine incontinence. Improving one's health and self-assurance can result from treating this issue.

THE END

www.ingramcontent.com/pod-product-compliance
Lightning Source LLC
Chambersburg PA
CBHW070048260726
48658CB00002B/784